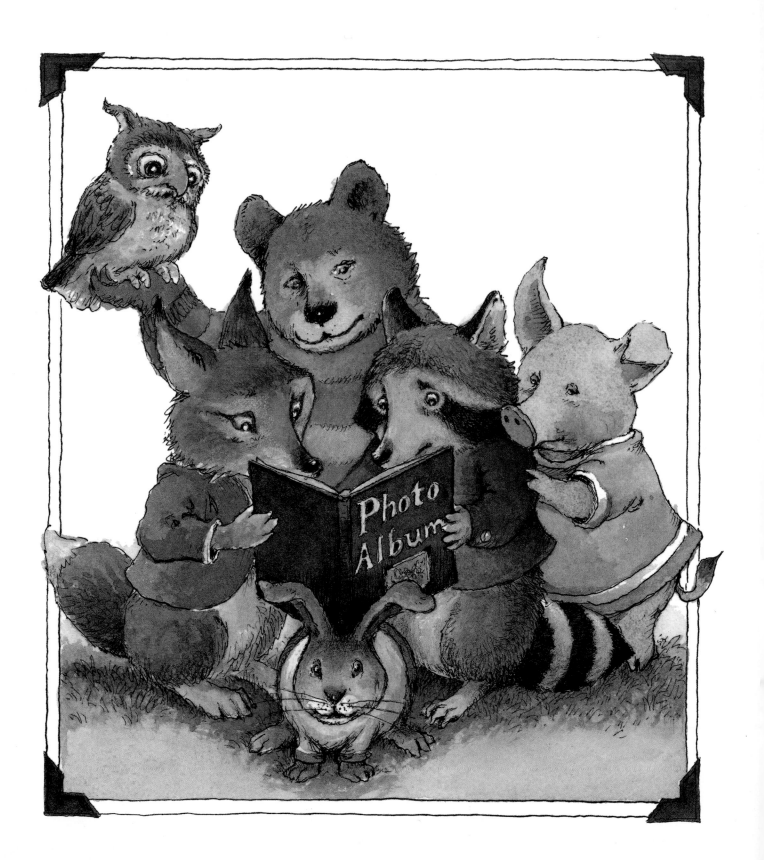

The Hope Tree

♥

KIDS TALK ABOUT BREAST CANCER

WRITTEN BY Laura Numeroff AND Wendy S. Harpham, M.D.

ILLUSTRATIONS BY David McPhail

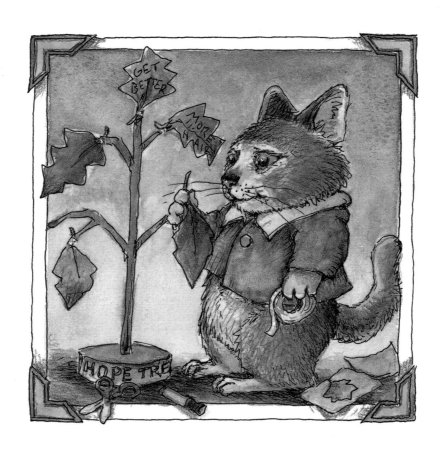

SIMON & SCHUSTER BOOKS FOR YOUNG READERS

New York • London • Toronto • Sydney • Singapore

For all women everywhere, for their courage—L. N.
For all children who love someone with cancer—W. S. H.
For Laura, a good sport always—D. M.

A Note on *The Hope Tree*

The Hope Tree was created to help families talk about the difficult issues of breast cancer in healthy and hopeful ways. Drawn from real stories about mothers with cancer, *The Hope Tree* focuses on ten key topics that often affect families dealing with illness. Animal characters in an imaginary support group are used to provide insights and advice in a comforting format.

SIMON & SCHUSTER BOOKS FOR YOUNG READERS

An imprint of Simon & Schuster Children's Publishing Division
1230 Avenue of the Americas, New York, New York 10020

Text copyright © 1999 by Laura Numeroff and Wendy S. Harpham, M.D.
Illustrations copyright © 1999 by David McPhail
The Hope Tree: Kids Talk About Breast Cancer was originally published as *Kids Talk: Kids Speak Out About Breast Cancer*
by Samsung Telecommunications America and Sprint PCS.
The authors and illustrator thank Samsung and Sprint for their assistance with this new edition,
as well as Bill Smith Studio for all their help.
The authors and illustrator have donated all of their royalties from this book to the Susan G. Komen Breast Cancer Foundation.
Simon & Schuster Books for Young Readers has made a one-time donation as well.

Book design by Paula Winicur
The text for this book is set in Lomba.
The illustrations are rendered in watercolor over pencil.

Printed in Hong Kong
2 4 6 8 10 9 7 5 3
Library of Congress Cataloging-in-Publication Data
Numeroff, Laura Joffe.
The hope tree: kids talk about breast cancer / written by Laura Numeroff and Wendy S. Harpham; illustrated by David McPhail.
p. cm.
Summary: Various kids describe their feelings and how they cope with their mothers' breast cancer
ISBN 0-689-84526-X
[1.Breast—Cancer—Juvenile literature. 2.Children of cancer patients—Juvenile literature.]
I. Harpham, Wendy Schlessel. II. McPhail, David M., ill. III. Title
RC280.B8 .N86 2001
[E]—dc21
2001020332

ABOUT THE SUSAN G. KOMEN BREAST CANCER FOUNDATION

The story of the Susan G. Komen Breast Cancer Foundation begins in 1980, when Nancy Brinker lost her sister and best friend, Susan Goodman Komen, to breast cancer at the age of thirty-six. As Nancy watched her sister die, she wondered how this could happen in one of the most medically advanced countries in the world. Nancy made a promise to her sister: She would dedicate the rest of her life to making a difference for those who would face a breast cancer diagnosis. In 1982, she started the Susan G. Komen Breast Cancer Foundation to help that promise become a reality.

Twenty years ago, very few resources were available for young people looking for answers to questions too overwhelming to comprehend. Susan Komen's own two children, just like Nancy's young son when she was diagnosed with breast cancer in 1984, were frightened and confused when facing their mothers' illness. Fortunately, now there are resources like *The Hope Tree* to help children reach out and talk about those issues, to realize that there are others just like them experiencing these uncertainties.

Nancy Brinker established the Komen Foundation with only a few hundred dollars of her own and a shoe box full of friends' names. Today, the Komen Foundation is the largest private funding source for breast cancer research and community outreach programs. Since 1982, the Komen Foundation—along with more than 100 affiliates nationally, as well as in Greece, Germany, and Italy—has raised in excess of $300 million to support our mission: to eradicate breast cancer as a life-threatening disease by advancing research, education, screening, and treatment. Key to this success is the Komen Race for the Cure®, the largest series of 5K runs/fitness walks in the world. This event, created by Nancy, has grown from one local race with 800 participants to a national series with more than 1.3 million participants expected in 2001.

The Komen Foundation is thrilled to be involved with *The Hope Tree*. There is still far to go in the fight against breast cancer, but the support and help available today are greater than ever. We thank Laura, Wendy, and David for supporting the Komen Foundation with this wonderful book, and for their important contribution to the breast cancer effort.

—*Susan Braun*,
President and CEO

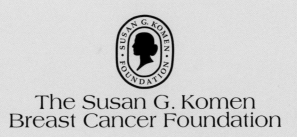

The Susan G. Komen
Breast Cancer Foundation

A NOTE TO YOU FROM US!

We all belong to a really cool group called KIDS TALK. Once a week we play games and talk about movies, our families, sports, school, books, and, oh yeah, our moms' cancer. You see, we share something in common: All of our moms have breast cancer.

This scrapbook will show you some of the things we went through. If your mom has breast cancer, maybe it will help you. We hope so!

Anthony, Emma, Lily, David, Sophie, Sarah,
Jamal, Miguel, Kisa and Kim, and Jessie

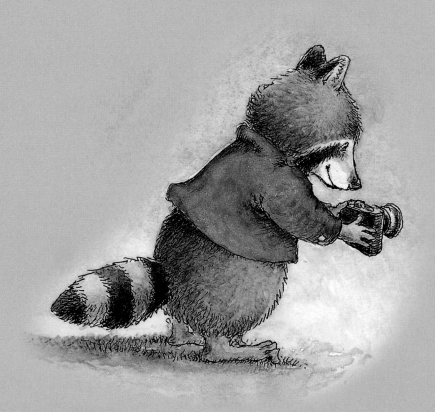

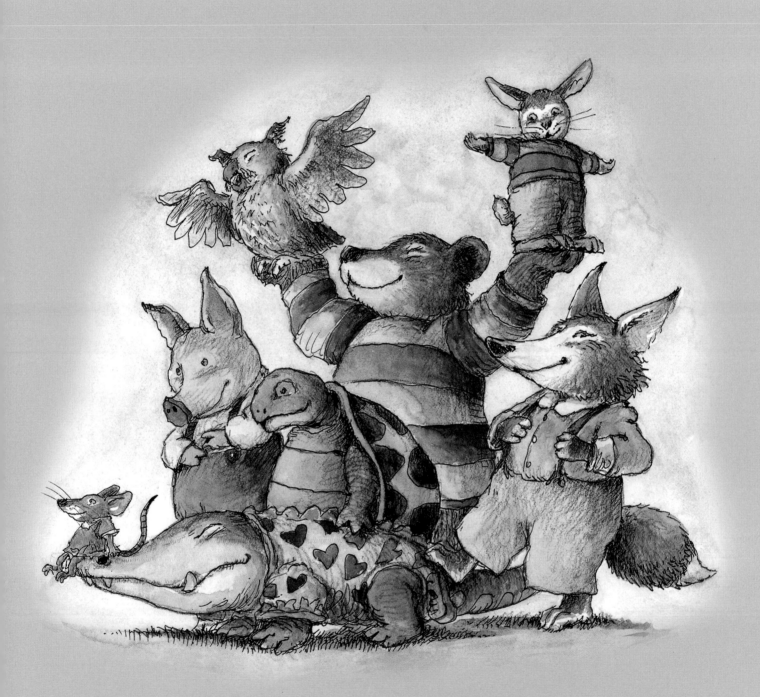

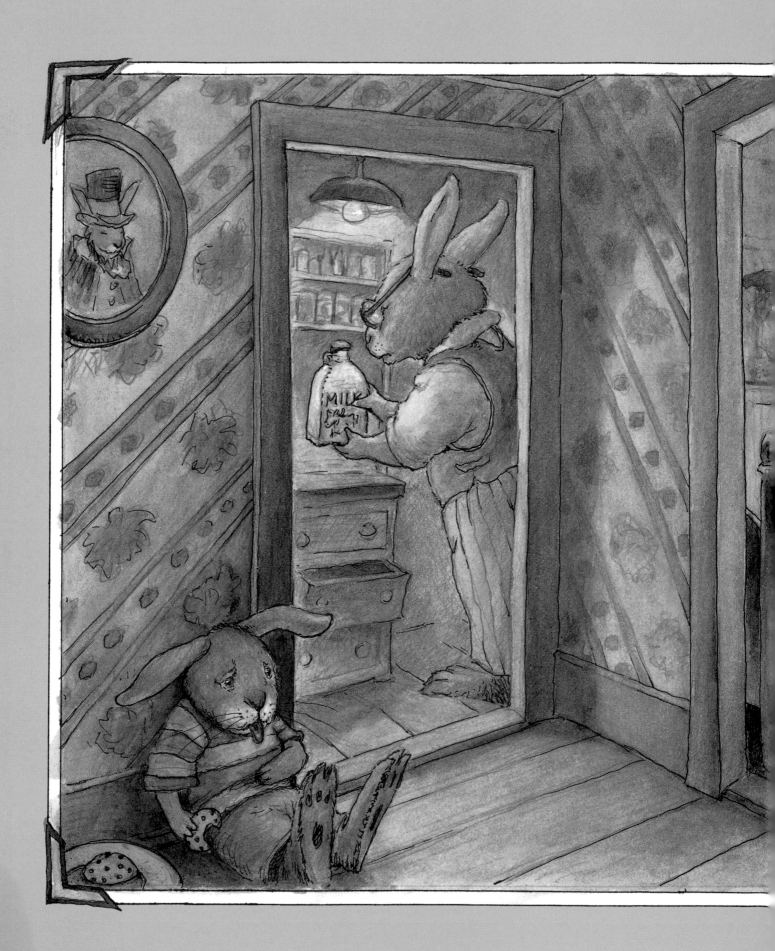

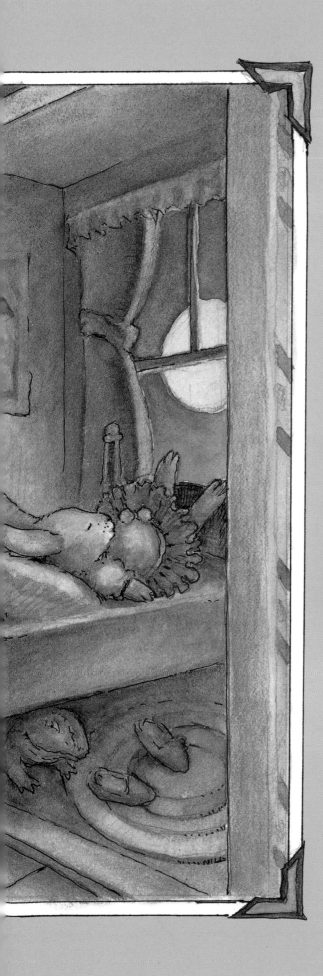

THE DAY MY FAMILY FOUND OUT

This is a picture from the day my family found out that my mom had breast cancer. Everything was so messed up. There were a gazillion phone calls, my mom and dad were whispering, and I even heard my mom crying. I wasn't sure what was going on, but I knew it wasn't good. I was scared.

Nothing got done that day. My mom didn't do the weekly grocery shopping (so I ate cookies for dinner!); my iguana, Sydney, got loose; my dad put milk in the pantry; and my sister went to sleep in her tutu. My house was never crazy like that before.

Anthony, age 8

PICTURING CANCER MAKES IT LESS SCARY

Cancer is hard to understand. All I know is that cancer is something that grows inside a person's body, but it's not supposed to be there.

I made a poster to show how cancer reminds me of weeds. You have to get rid of weeds, otherwise they keep growing and crowd out the flowers. Some weeds are easier to get rid of than others.

There are lots of different ways to get rid of weeds: pulling, cutting them, or using weed spray. Doctors use different ways to get rid of cancer: surgery, chemotherapy, radiation, and pills.

The first picture is filled with weeds. That's like when my mother had cancer. This next picture is my garden without any weeds—just beautiful flowers that are healthy and strong. And the last picture is my mom when her cancer is all gone.

Emma, age 10

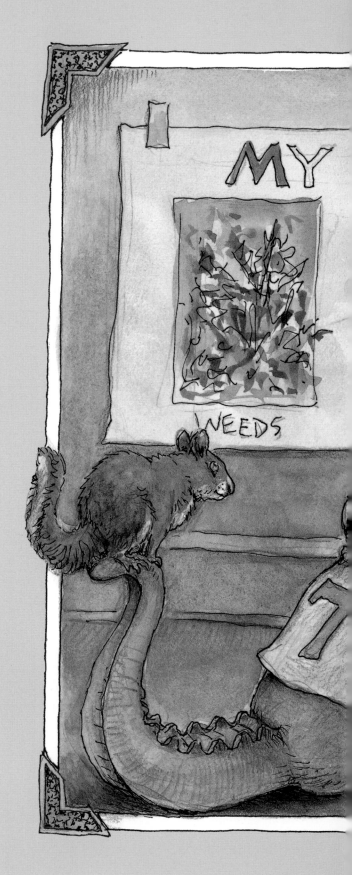

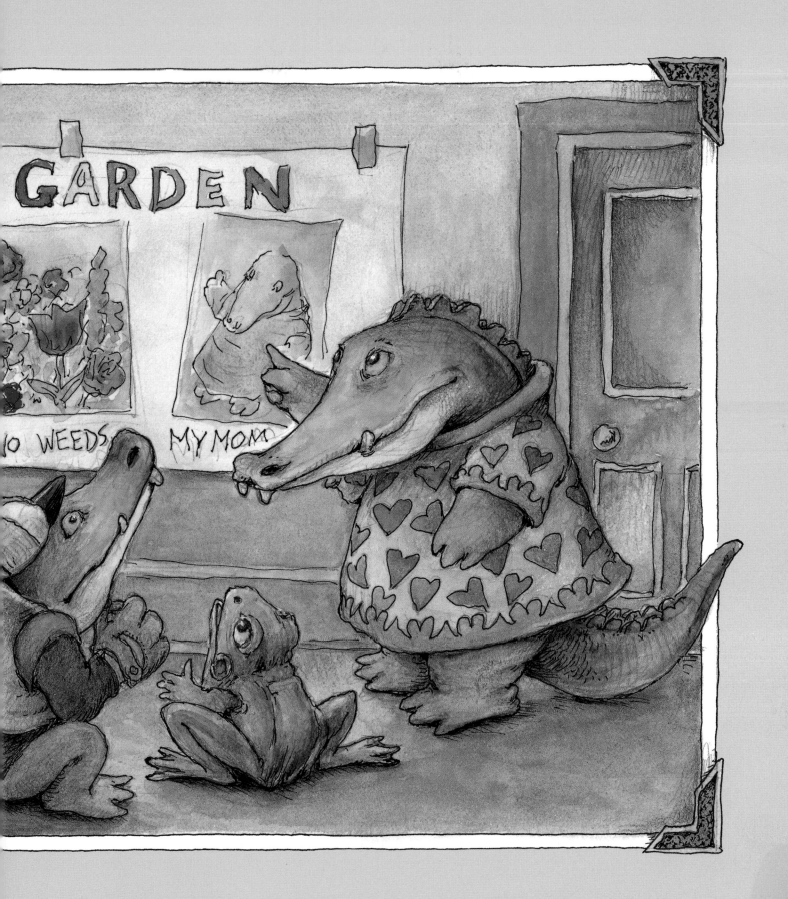

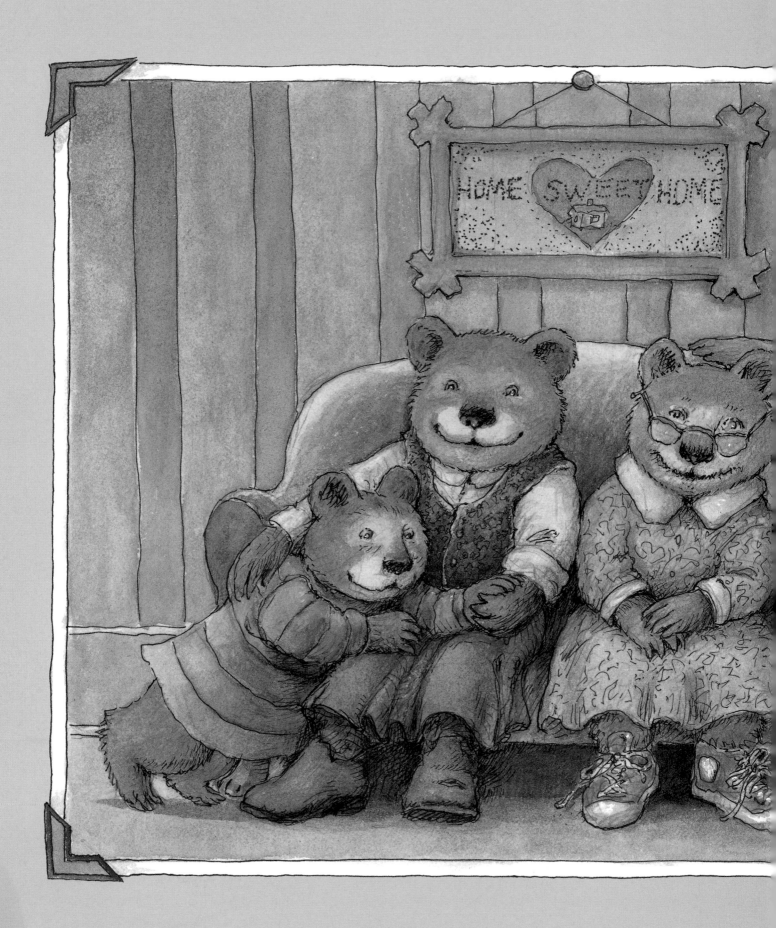

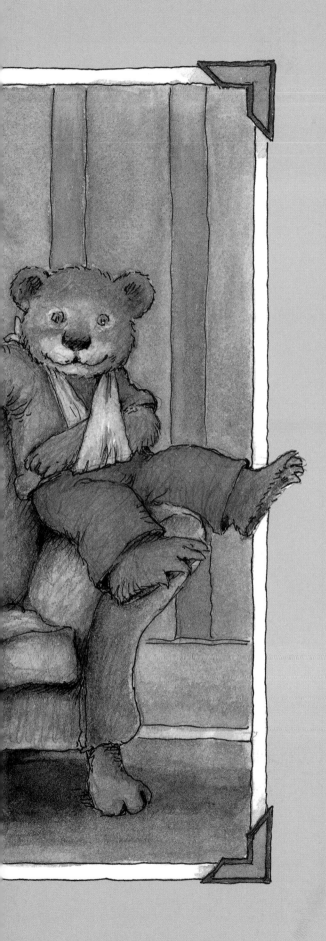

YOU CAN'T CATCH IT!

Boy, was I worried that I could catch my mom's cancer. But the doctor said, "Lily, there is NO WAY you can 'catch' your mom's cancer, just like there's NO WAY you can catch Trevor's broken arm."

Here's my mom, my grandma, my brother, and me. We could still scrunch close together for the picture because you can't catch broken arms or cancer from other people. I'm glad I can't catch cancer because I like hugging my mom.

But some days Mom is just too tired or hurts too much to snuggle. I made a "love phone" to send my hugs and kisses to my mom when I have to be careful of her owies. I use it for my grandma, too, but not for Trevor!

Lily, age 6

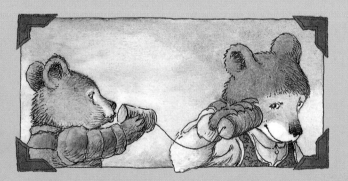

DOCTORS AND NURSES MAKE MOM BETTER

My brother (Jack), my stepbrothers (Simon and Spencer), my stepdad, and I visited the clinic where Mom gets her treatments. We looked at the equipment and asked all of our questions. Simon asked if we could take one of the IV poles home! He's only four.

The nice people at the clinic are doing everything possible to help Mom feel better and get her well again. They even gave us bandages and little flashlights to keep. It was really neat.

David, age 7 $\frac{1}{2}$

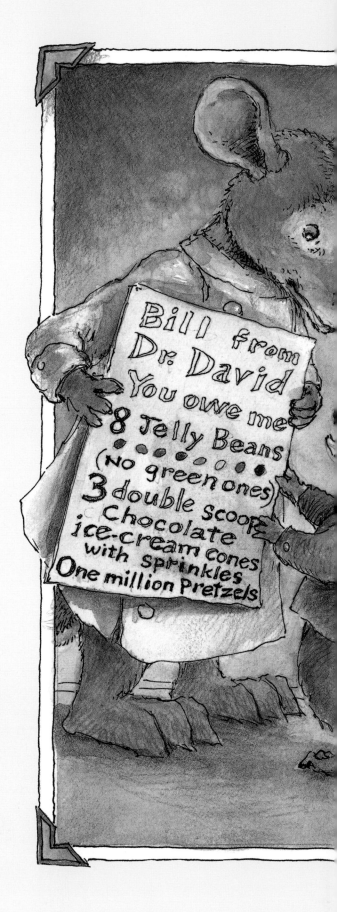

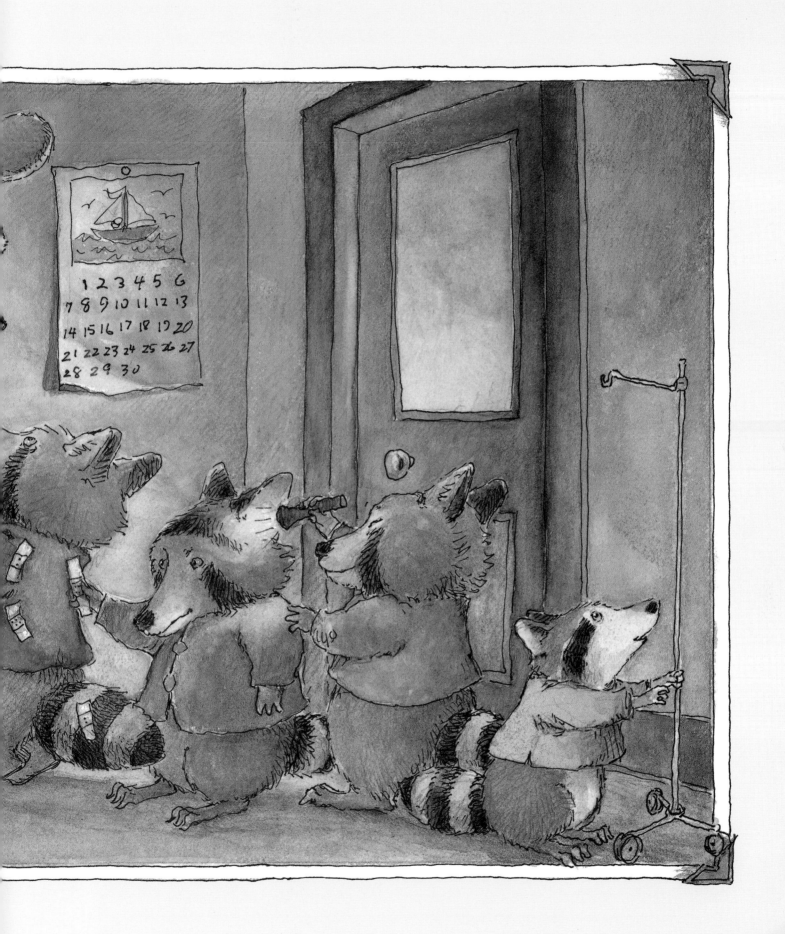

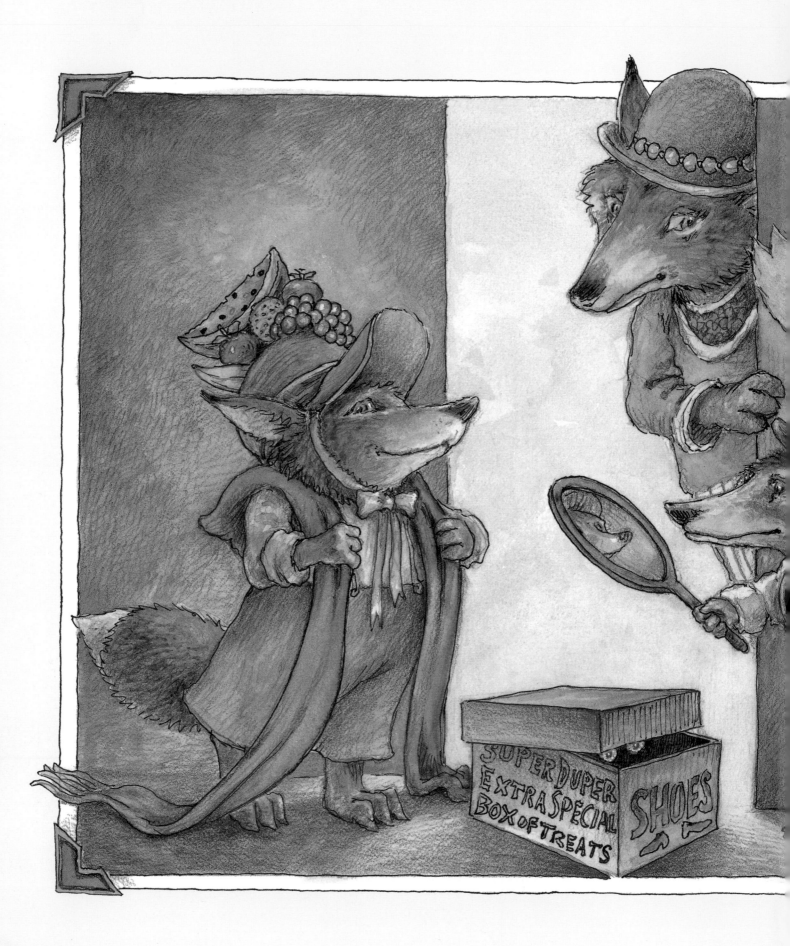

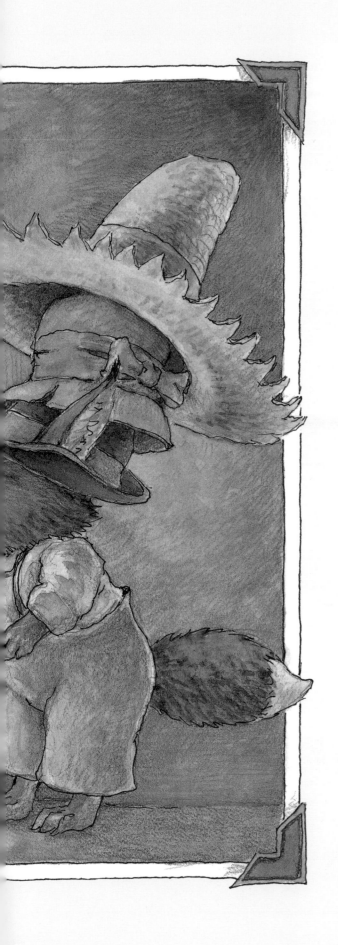

LOOKING FOR GOOD THINGS IN THE CHANGES

Here's my twin, Katie, and me playing dress-up. Mom got a whole bunch of scarves and hats because the chemo made her hair fall out. I don't like that Mom is bald. I get soooo embarrassed in front of my friends, even when she wears her hats and scarves. But Mom keeps reminding me that she's bald because the medicine is working. That's good.

Another thing that bugs me are the days Mom gets her chemo. First she's gone most of the day, then she comes home tired and cranky. Katie and I found a way to cheer up on chemo days: We decorated Katie's biggest shoe box and filled it with fun toys, books, and some surprises! The rule is we can only open our special box on the days Mom has chemo.

I put in a special surprise for Katie . . . I can't wait until she finds it!

Sophie, age 7

LOOK FOR THE GOOD IN SOMETHING BAD

This is my family at last year's big picnic! We usually go to a park far from home, but that day my mom was too tired. She looked sad. So, we filled the bathtub and called it Lake Scrubatub. We had an awesome time. And there were no ants!

I learned that when your mom has cancer, one thing you CAN expect is that there will be some bad days. When bad things happen because of Mom's cancer, we all try really hard to turn them into good things. Sometimes we can't. But we always try our very best. This helps us feel better. And Mom feels better, too!

Sarah, age 5

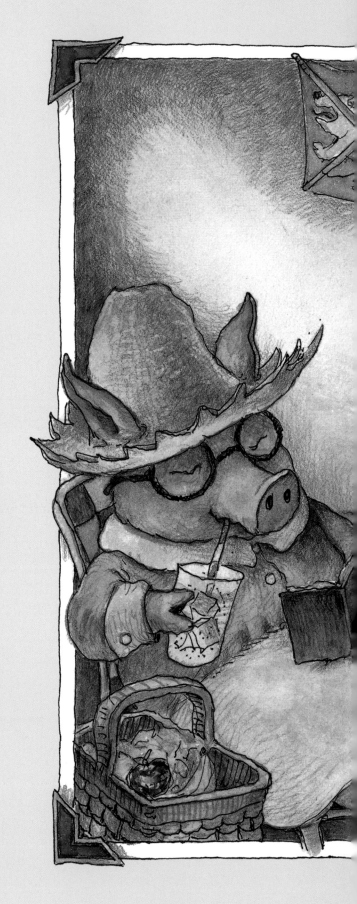

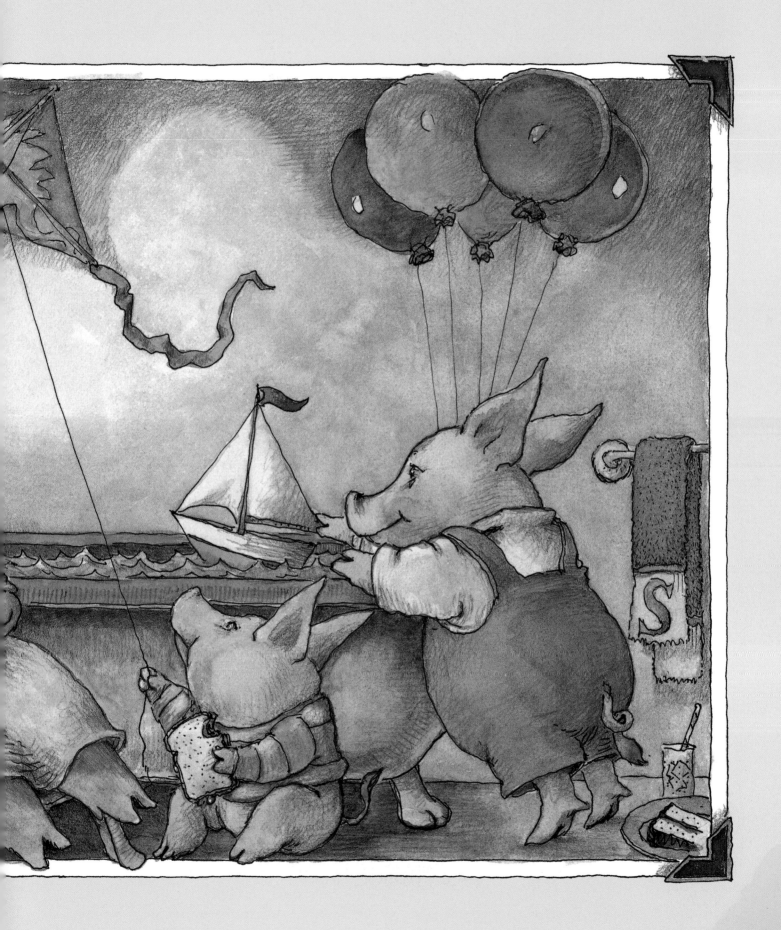

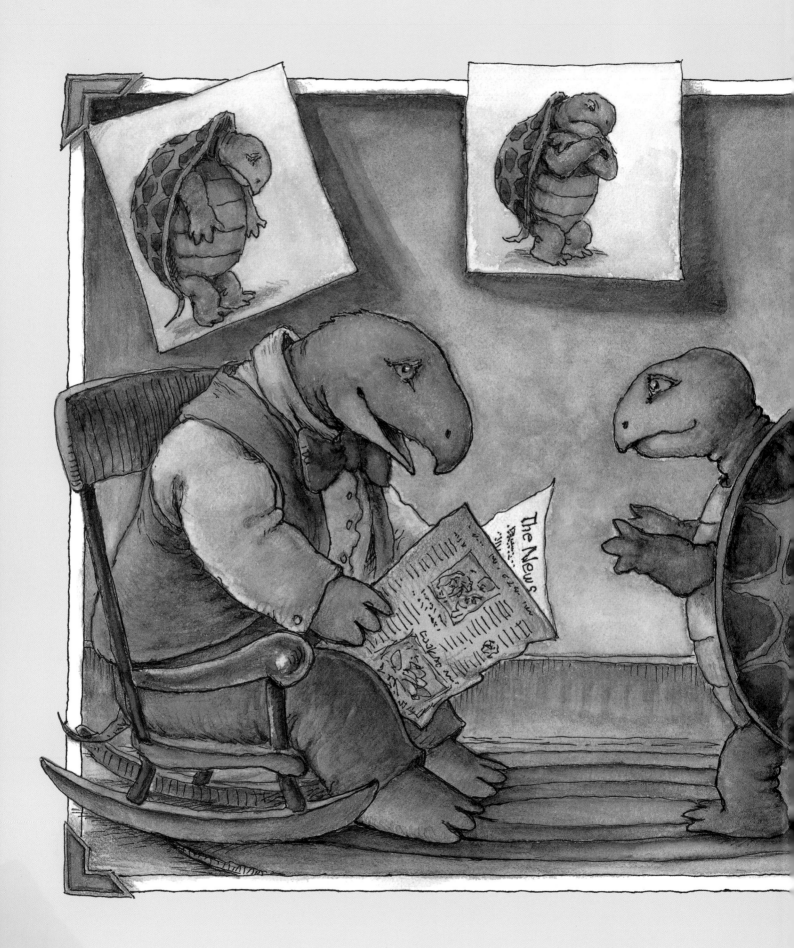

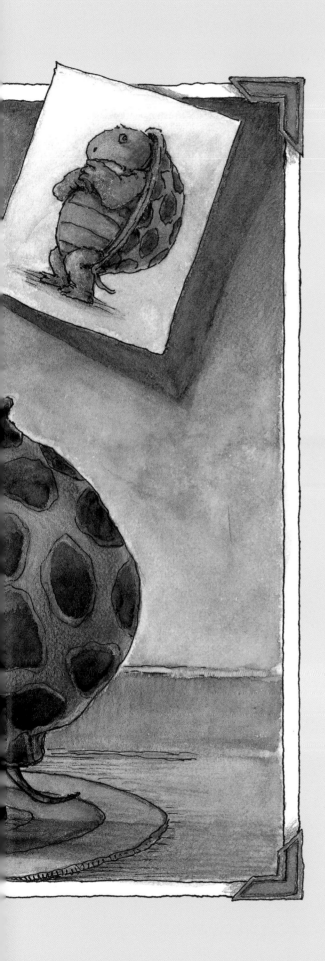

AN OCEAN OF EMOTION

This is my grandpop. He listens to me when I feel down. I've been having a whole bunch of yucky feelings since my mom got cancer.

First, I was really sad. Then I got mad about all the changes. I was so worried her cancer was my fault, but Grandpop promised me it wasn't. I believe him because he's a very smart man. (I hope I'm as smart as he is when I grow up.)

I talk about how I feel with my friends from school, too, and with my new friends at KIDS TALK. Now I know it's also okay to feel happy about other things even when my mom is feeling crummy.

Whatever we feel doesn't change the most important thing: We all want our moms to get better! As soon as possible!

Jamal, age 12

FAMILY MEETINGS

This picture is from one of my family's meetings. We sure needed them after my mom started treatment. Before, everyone argued about who was allowed to do what, and I never knew what I was supposed to do.

Meetings help everyone in my family talk to one another: Mom and Dad explain the new rules, like who takes out the garbage or who puts the dishes in the sink. (I'd rather put the dishes in the sink!) Talking with my family helps me understand what's going on and makes me feel better and a lot less lonely. Now I feel like we're all on the same team!

You don't have to have special meet-ings to talk, but if you do, you might end them with a snack. We like peanut butter chip cookies!

Miguel, age 7

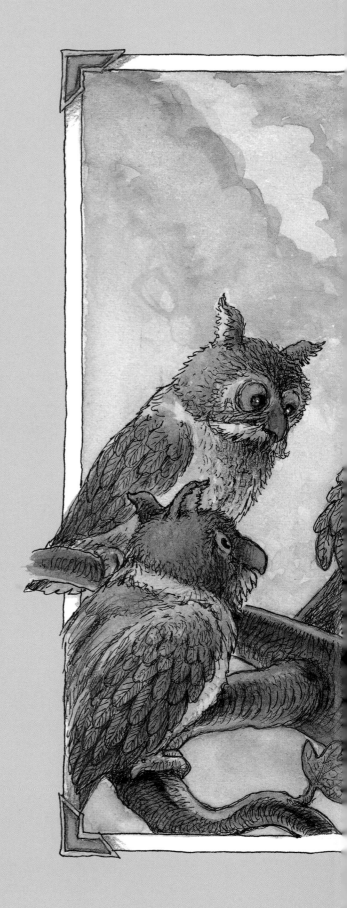

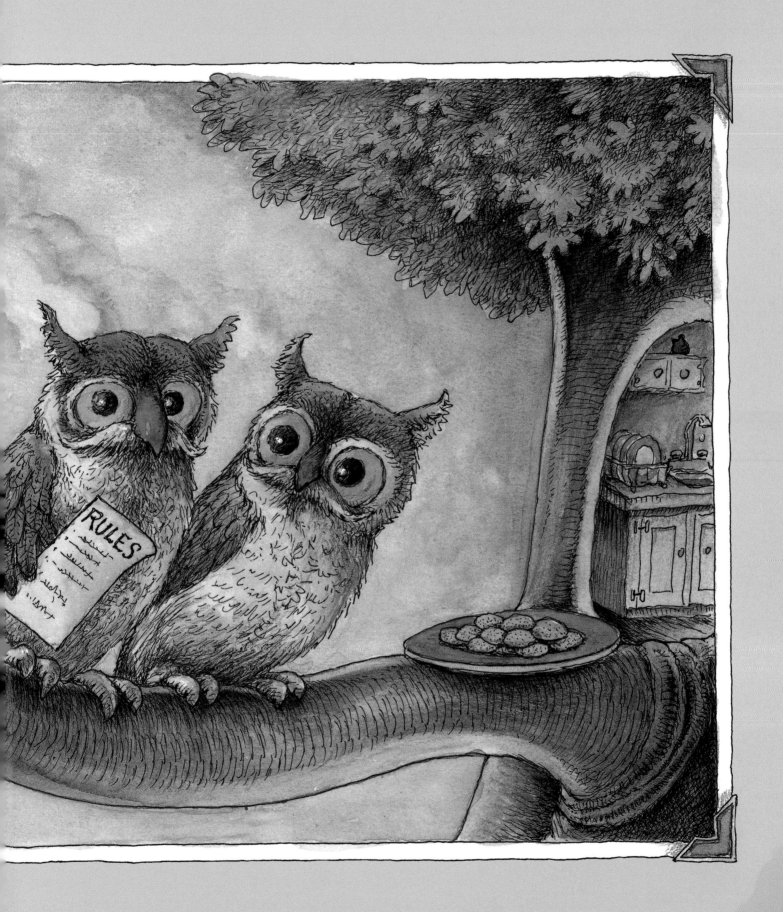

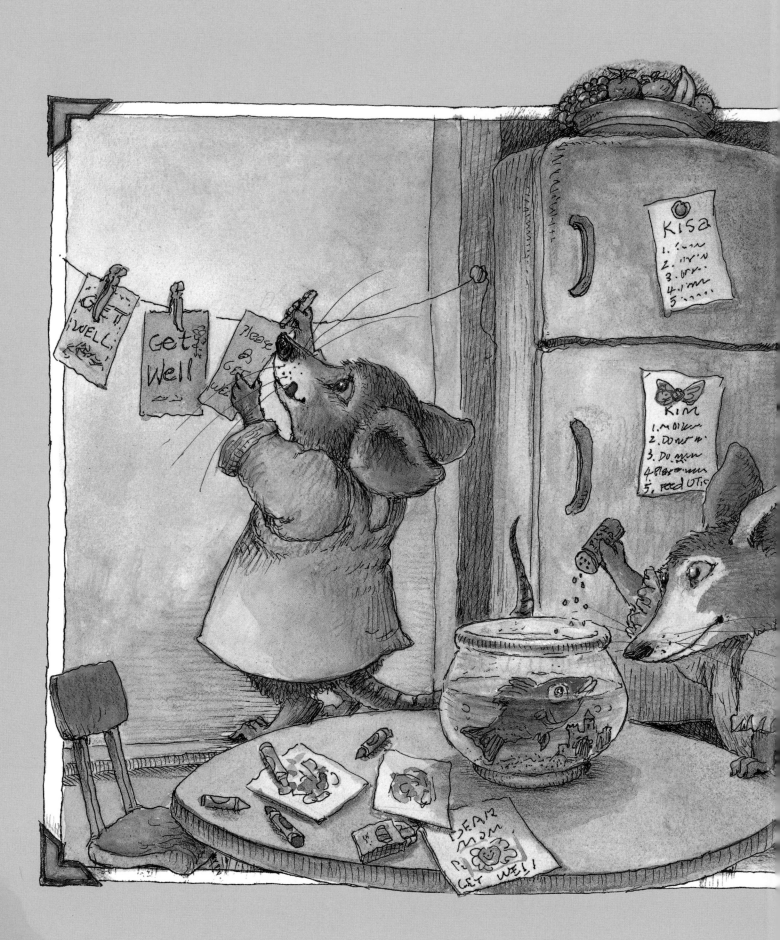

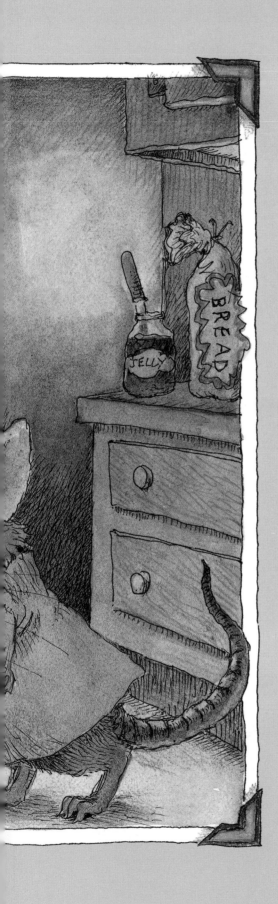

HELPING HELPS

We sure wish we could fix our moms' cancer.

Even though we can't, there are lots of things we CAN do to help out. Here are our lists:

Kisa
1. Hang up all the get well cards
2. Make pictures to cheer up Mom
3. Pick up my room
4. Don't tease Kim
5. Work hard in kindergarten

Kim
1. Make my lunch
2. Don't tease Kisa
3. Do my best at school
4. Play quietly while Mom naps
5. Feed Otis

Kim, age 8
Kisa, age 5½

THE HOPE TREE

At every meeting of KIDS TALK, we all share stories about having hope. Some of us pray, and that helps. Jamal talks to his grandpop. My big sister writes in her diary. (I'm not allowed to peek.)

Miguel's mom visited our group after her hair grew back, and she was all healthy again. That helped me feel hopeful.

Even when I'm scared, or my mom is very sick, I can still have hope: hope for her to get all better; hope for her to have a good day; and hope for me to feel less afraid, too.

This is my hope tree. I write on each paper leaf something I am hoping for. Some leaves stay the same. Other leaves change. When a wish comes true, or when something I hope for doesn't happen, I make a new leaf with a new hope.

Keep hoping.

Jessie, age 9 $\frac{1}{2}$

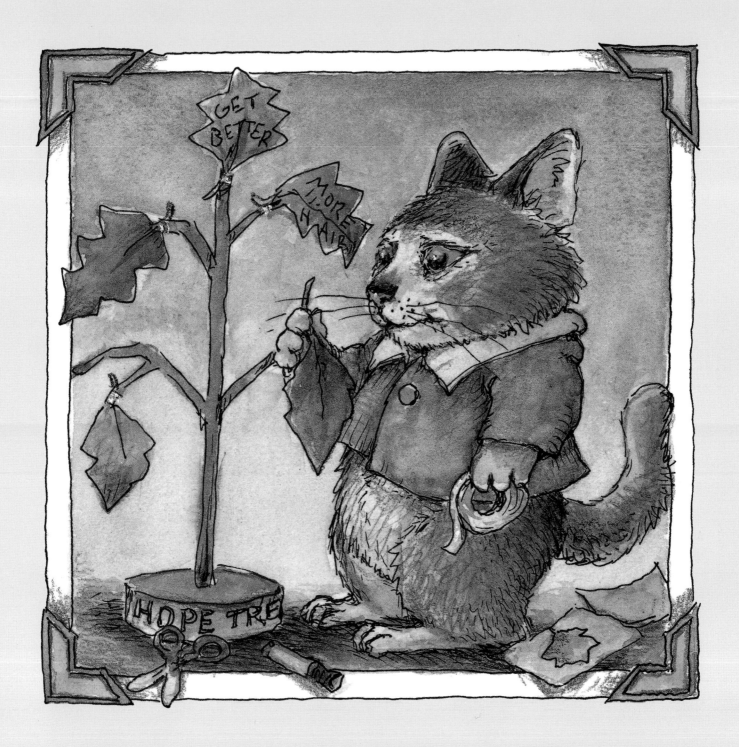